Tales of Perimenopause & Aging from a Middle-Age Around the Way Girl

By Kathy M. Henry

Dedications

This book is dedicated to my fabulous daughters, Nu-Nu and Boogie. I am telling my story so that they will not be as clueless as I was and still am during this stage in their lives when it comes. This book is also dedicated to all the other sisters around the world who are struggling with perimenopause and aging in society that worships youth. We go make it, we go make it!!!

Preface

Perimenopause is a term I learned about in 2003. I was bleeding excessively during my periods on a regular basis (had fibroids and it took 13 years for me to find out and another two years to get treatment because no one listens to Black women), was surfing the internet, and clicked on an article about this phenomena. Now why did I think my almost 33 year old ass was going through perimenopause at that time I will never know but when I went to my ob-gyn, I got shot down quickly. It is so ironic that he couldn't be bothered to check for fibroids but he knew I wasn't going through perimenopause but as usual, I am digressing.

Perimenopause can be described as the season before menopause actually happens. Menopause is the cessation if the menstrual cycle in a woman's life and perimenopause is the staircase that women must climb in order to achieve menopause. And it is a raggedy ass staircase filled with holes and empty 40 ounce bottles.

So this short e-book will be about my own personal journey during this very special time in a woman's life. I have been dealing with perimenopause for six years and it has been a bumpy ride y'all. It will also discuss the challenges women face in a society that worship youth and put the elders in the pasture. Especially women.

Society has really brainwashed people into believing that getting older as a woman is a fate worse than death. And although I am just a peon in this world, I have to add my voice to dismantling this bullshit. Becoming a Crone has been the most freeing experience I've ever encountered in the almost 52 years I've been alive and I want other women to experience this feeling of liberation from societal expectations. This complete joy in knowing that you are still alive and thriving despite the anti-older woman propaganda.

I hope to educate and amuse people with my journey. Enjoy folks.

Disclaimer

These are the symptoms I have experienced while going through perimenopause but every woman on this planet is different so your symptoms might be totally different than mine. Hell, you might not have any symptoms at all but do not try to blame me for anything that you are experiencing or might experience. I make no claims to be a doctor; I'm just a middle-age, fat around the way girl from the South East Side of Chicago.

Table Of Contents

PERIMENOPAUSE SYMPTOMS

Pimples

Perimenopause began for me the summer of 2016. It during this time when I noticed that I kept breaking out with pimples located on my cheeks, along my jaw line, under my chin area. Big ugly ass pimples, red and painful and when I busted the fuckers, scars would form.

Now being an adult, I should have known better than to pick at my face but the 14-year-old girl that I used to be is still deeply entrenched within me and she could not help herself. So as result, I looked fucked up for a minute so I started using foundation. The scars would eventually go away but this constant breakout of pimples made me do some research online and voila! I rediscovered perimenopause.

Perimenopause causes hormonal changes in a woman's body because her estrogen levels are dropping. The ovaries are the producers of estrogen and as a woman gets older, the ovaries don't produce as much estrogen because the baby factor is about to shut down. The ovaries also produce progesterone and combined, they are the hormones responsible for periods and ovulation, the wicked heifers. A better description of this process is in the link below:

https://my.clevelandclinic.org/health/ diseases/21608-perimenopause.

I was 45 at the time and although I wasn't surprised, I was quite annoyed. We as women are always going through some shit with our bodies and it seems like we can't ever get a break. Weight gain, acne breakouts, hormonal issues, hot flashes, and emotional highs from the mountaintop to emotional lows in the gutter, I have experienced it all in the last six years. And frankly, I am sick of this shit. I had a red pimple on my top lip a few weeks ago that looked like I sucked the wrong peenie-weenie when I haven't had sexual relations with a man in almost three years. The hormonal imbalance is a true bitch y'all.

Weight Gain

I have lost and gained probably 75 pounds these past six years. On New Year's Day 2016, I had plans to cook fried catfish, smothered potatoes, cabbage, and baked salmon. Then I got on the scale and learned that I was almost at 300 pounds. Menu plans changed very quickly and all the fish got baked, and the potatoes got baked.

Until the end of year, I had baked chicken and cabbage several times per week and I lost almost 60 pounds. Not quite high school skinny but I was looking good. Then by the end of year, the weight started creeping back like the trifling fucker it is and I decided do Keto starting in 2017. Lost 5 pounds that first week of 2017 and then I gained 7 pounds the following week. And ever since then, the battle to lose weight has been on because those hormones I mentioned earlier that causes pimple outbreaks also makes it hard to lose weight. Perimenopause will have your self-esteem in the gutter thinking that you are less than nothing because you cannot lose 10 pounds although you are eating dust.

During the pandemic, I gained 35 pounds and was officially over the 300 pound mark. I was a real big girl. A big, big girl. Two tons of fun and all that good shit. You should have seen the look on my face at the doctor's office when I was prescribed diabetic and high blood medication. I was like "hell nah" and made up my mind to get those 35 pounds off my ass.

 And I did but I cannot get below 250 pounds for shit and it is makes my ass itch and twitch. Especially when people who have never had a weight problem in their lives decide to give you unsolicited "advice" on how to lose weight. Like go sit your boney ass down somewhere and hush. Yes I am being rude and probably will be accused of "skinny shaming" on the social media but I do not give a fuck or a rat's ass. Until you step into my shoes as a middle age, fat woman going through hormonal changes due to Mother Nature, you cannot tell me anything so fuck you.

I am currently working outside the home so I am getting my exercise on and eating balanced meals but

I still cannot lose any weight to save my life. The upside is that I have not gained any weight which is a good thing because at least something good has come out of this madness. And the greatest thing about this weight loss battle over the past six years is that it has truly taught me to love myself whether I am big as a house or small as a cute, little kitten. So this aspect of perimenopause has been good for me mentally because I struggled for years dealing with being a plus size woman in a culture that hates all women but hold a particular contempt for the larger variety of women. Now these folks can't tell me shit. Fuck them all.

Hot Flashes

I have talked to girlfriends who are catching hell with the hot flashes, having to change their sheets nightly because of the sweating but I have been lucky so. Because although I get hot flashes, I don't sweat; it just feels like I am going to burst into a puff of smoke like Mr. Twiddle from that Tex Avery cartoon "Sh-h-h-h-h-h." My electricity bill increases faithfully every summer because the air conditioner in my boudoir is on full blast. So to all my sisters who sweating like you ran in a marathon but is merely sitting on the couch, my heart goes out to y'all.

Periods

My periods during this era were hellish. I had fibroids but I did not know this when I started perimenopause and my monthly flow had become so heavy and complete with blood clots that I had to use tampons and two pads. Sometimes three pads. I had to call off during the beginning of my menstrual cycle because I just could not make to work the first two days. Some months, I would bleed for weeks at a time. Weeks, not days but weeks.

I learned that I had fibroids in November of 2018 when an ultrasound was performed on me. The technician found a huge mass in my uterus and immediately, my gynecologist decided to make sure the mass was not cancerous so a test was taken. Waiting to receive the results was one of the scariest times ever but I was one of the lucky ones because the fibroids were benign.

My gynecologist wanted to perform a hysterectomy on me but I was not feeling that at all because I have been getting cut on since I was 16-years-old. I have had three c-sections, and an ectopic pregnancy in which the right fallopian tube was removed. But fate would step in a few months later.

I had developed a hacking cough and decided to go Northwestern Memorial Hospital before I went to work in February of 2019. While there, I was asked by the receptionist did I have any other health conditions and I told her about the fibroids. She gave my information to the gynecology department;

a nurse called me and set up an appointment to get another ultrasound, more tests to see if the fibroids were cancerous, and then an appointment with the fella who would change my life: Dr. Chris who performed a procedure on me called uterine fibroid embolization.

It is completely noninvasive way to make fibroids go away. The procedure was performed on March 28, 2019, my youngest daughter's 18th birthday and since the procedure was performed, my life drastically changed for the better. I still had periods but the heavy bleeding and blood clots stopped completely. Lately I have not had a period at all praise Jesus and all his apostles. I could actually live a normal life for a little bit.

Emotional Thunderstorms, Tornados, & Whirlwinds

Estrogen and progesterone, the hormones produced by the ovaries that causes the menstrual cycle and wrecks havoc in women as we age also causes our emotions to show their asses during the aging process. As a woman who is emotional by nature, filled with passion and fire, this aspect of perimenopause has been kicking my ass full throttle.

How can I explain this aspect clearly? I will be watching a Bugs Bunny cartoon and memories will flood my heartwhen I was a little girl waiting for my mother to wake up on a Saturday morning to make me some scrambled eggs and I will start crying. Full fledge tears complete with snot flying and red eyes. Then five minutes later, I am cackling madly at Yosemite Sam getting his ass kicked.

Over the past six years, I have lost so many family and friends to the specter of death. My cousins Jerome and Jeremy who died in 2016 and 2017. Jerome was the same age as me and he would come to Chicago every summer after his mother Joe-Ann moved to San Francisco. He was my summer brother and I loved him. When he died from diabetes complications, I was devastated.

Jeremy was my cousin's Lisa son and he was three years older than my eldest daughter so I loved him of a combination of a little brother, cousin and son all wrapped up into one. He died at the age of 33 from heart issues and it was a complete shock to the family.

Earlier in 2017 before Jeremy crossed over, I had lost two friends back to back, Chuckie and Charnette. I grew up with them, hung out with them and I loved them. Chuckie and I lived on the same block and all the girls had a crush on him because he was fine as hell but he didn't pay any attention to us because he knew we were too young for him. Charnette lived on the next block and she treated me like a little sister.

In 2018, my world came crashing down when my

cousin Cleo died. She was technically a first cousin by blood but she was more than that to me. She was a big sister, aunt, and a mother figure after my mother died in 2006. Going to her funeral was one the hardest days in my life and to be frank, her death was harder on me than my mother's because I had really convinced myself that she would live forever.

On December 7, 2019, I received a phone call and learned that my friend Trena had died from a heart ailment. She was only 45 years old and whew. She was just not a friend but my sister. This year would have been the 30th anniversary of our friendship and I still cannot believe that my friend is gone forever.

In 2020, an entire chapter in my life ended when my brother Larry died because with his death, I became the sole survivor of my mother's branch of the family tree. My mother gave birth to three children and I am the only one who is left. It has been a heavy burden to bear but I am coping, at times barely.

Last year, I lost two more friends that I grew up with, Genial and Mikki. Genial died in June of 2021 and Mikki died two months later in August. We spent our teens, 20s, 30s, 40s, and I was hoping our 50s together but it wasn't meant to be unfortunately.

I am sure people will wonder why I am speaking of my lost ones while discussing perimenopause but I just want people to know what I have been dealing with emotionally over the past six years in addition to dealing with the hormonal changes caused by perimenopause. In a different decade, I would have been put in an insane asylum for women because of the tears I have shed.

I believe that I would have grieved for my people just as hard if they had crossed over when I was a younger woman but the hormonal changes in my body these past few years has made the grieving process worse. My hair has turned almost silver in the past three years and I have permanent dark mark on the sides of my eyes because of the tears I have shed. I went into grief therapy and it helped immensely but these hormones are still whupping my ass emotionally and sometimes, I just want to crawl up in a ball and stare at a wall for the rest of my life. I can't do that and I have to keep moving and I have. But life stepped in again and had to deal with a major league health issue.

I got diagnosed with epilepsy in October of 2020.

Had my first seizure a month before my 49th birthday and was officially diagnosed as an epileptic a month before my 50th. I am such a special person aren't I (said with much sarcasm)? Now I am on anti-seizure medication that makes me tired from dawn to dusk and still dealing with perimenopause. If I was a weaker individual, I would have had a nervous breakdown but in spite of all the pain and trauma I have experienced these past six years, I am eternally grateful to be still alive and have most of my brain power still intact. Nothing or no one is going to break me.

16

LET'S TALK ABOUT WHY THIS TOPIC IS SO TABOO AMONGST BLACK WOMEN

Foolishness From Your Own Kind

I am a feminist by the way and have been one for 25 years. In the words of a great woman named Maya Angelo, "I'm a feminist. I've been a female for a long time now. It'd be stupid not to be on my own side." But some of us are just that stupid and have passed down the stupidity to the next generation of women. A large part of this stupidity makes it almost impossible for us to have discussions with other women concerning our bodily functions. Too busy trying to look like invincible good girls who don't bleed monthly, don't have vaginal discharge like the rest of those other "dirty" women and all kinds of foolishness.

I get it, I really do. The Black church has done a complete mind job on the psyches of Black women and has been doing it for centuries. Shaming them for having a period in the first place, for having sexual desires, for merely existing but it is almost 2023. If you can find information on the internet on how to cast a spell on an errant boyfriend, you can find information about your body.

Like last year I was on Facebook and a friend had shared the status of a Black woman who announced her stupidity quite proudly to the world by writing that Black men's sperm was the determining factor on whether a biracial child was considered Black. If a Black woman had a child with a White man, that child is considered biracial but if it is the other way around, that child is considered Black. Yes y'all, she wrote this mess and it was a pack of ninnies agreeing with her. Now how can a woman with that mentality be of any use to another woman who is going through perimenopause or any other issue going on with her reproductive system? Just as useless as a turtle on its back.

How To Help Those Who Just Don't Know Any Better

So how do Black women like me and others fight this madness, this ignorance? To be quite honest, I do not know but I am hoping that this little e-book will be a start. I am always in these Black social media streets and I seldom see Black women discussing anything to do with our bodies other losing weight to get attention from men (never about health, all about that dick). All conversations are centered on men.

How to get a man, how to keep a man, how to find a new man if the last one leaves. Dick, dick, dick. For those reasons, I decided to write this book. I want Black women to stop feeling ashamed of being born female. To stop thinking that having a period, going through perimenopause, and eventually menopause is not normal because the church said so. We have take control of our own lives and stop letting outside facts such as men, society, churches, and other women determine our self-worth. I truly believe that once Black women come to this realization, their lives would change for the better.

EMBRACING THE CRONE

My perimenopausal journey has been hellish but it hopefully, it is coming to an end. I have not had a period since April and I am hoping that the bitch is gone for good because this year was the 40th anniversary of when my period started. It was June 26, 1982 and I was 11-years-old. I was playing with my Barbie dolls and watching Young and the Restless (when Terry Lester was still playing the role of Jack with his fine ass) and felt wetness down below. I put my hand down there and came up with blood, and my life has not been the same since. I know that some cultures embrace the start of the menstrual cycle but fuck that bitch.

When I know for a fact that my period has ceased, I am throwing a menopause party. It will be a bonfire consisting of empty Tampax and Kotex boxes and all my lady friends and I will dance around it, rejoicing that another sister has officially become a Crone. All my favorite foods will be served and we will listen to my favorite music all night long to the break of dawn.

Sex And The Perimenopausal Woman

My sex life used to be popping. Getting older changed something in me and it was for the better. I am a

Scorpio and Scorpios are considered the horniest out of all the zodiac signs and its true (giggle snort) but I had some shame issues as a Black, plus sized woman.

Black women are supposed to keep their legs closed but at the same time, suck dick on command. We are supposed to spin on that dick like a top spinner toy but remain chaste and pure in order to catch that high-value husband of our dreams.

And don't be a big girl because we are made to feel like absolute horse shit. I used to a wear nightgown when I was having an intimate interlude because I was ashamed of my body but not anymore. If you want to fuck me, you are going to accept these soft, lush rolls, the stretch marks on my belly that has given birth to three generations and if you don't like it, you can get the fuck on.

Perimenopause swept all those insecurities in the trash and I still have stalkers looking for this seasoned coochie but I have decided that it's not worth it. Read below.

A few paragraphs ago, I mentioned that my sex life used to be popping but I have been on an almost three year hiatus from sexual activity and I can't believe my horn dog ass has gone this long from some dick.

But in today's dating scene, it is quite easy to be celibate because these dudes expect a lot from women while looking like shit on stick. At this point in my life, I don't have much to give a man except for some pussy and men are some needy creatures. They need sex, food, therapy and a multitude of other things from women and I ain't got shit. Especially while going through perimenopause and these mood swings I be having. I don't want to end up in jail for busting a fella upside his head so in the meanwhile; all I do is dress and rest.

The Art Of Truly Not Giving A Fuck

Perimenopause and the death of my brother two years ago have changed me forever. I look at life through a totally different lens and I just don't give a fuck about too much anymore except the people that I love. At times, it scares me how little I care but for the most part, the joy of not giving a fuck has been freeing.

I no longer give a fuck about the opinions of others and everyone can kiss my fat, saggy ass. I will continue to wear loud, gaudy eye shadow in shades of electric blue, purple passion, and orange with matching eye liner to emphasize these slanty, sultry eyes of mine.

I will wear low cut dresses showing all of my glory and if you don't like what you see, turn your head and close your eyes. I have embraced the silver in my hair with pride instead of shame and my locs look luscious and wild, just like me. Embracing the wild ass Crone within has been a game changer.

Beginnings, Endings, And Something In The Middle

I truly hope that reading this short little book about my perimenopause journey helps my fellow sisters on how to be prepared for when their journey starts and educate the fellas who have mothers, girlfriends, and wives who are dealing with this issue. We as women have to stop walking around riddled with guilt for aging because aging is a privilege and nothing to be ashamed of. Learn to embrace the Crone ladies because she's a bad bitch. Aging is a gift, not a curse. Surround yourself with friends and family who love you and you will be okay.

I want to emphasis that these are the physical and emotional issues I have experienced during this time in my life and not every woman will have the same issues as I. Women are not all the same physically but those hormonal changes are real and I want women to be ready. One door opens with the start of the menstrual cycle and another one closes when menopause begins. Just look at perimenopause as the hallway between both journeys.

EPILOGUE

If Black women loved themselves with every inch of their beings, we would rule the world. Life doesn't end as you get older my sisters.

ABOUT THE AUTHOR

Kathy M. Henry

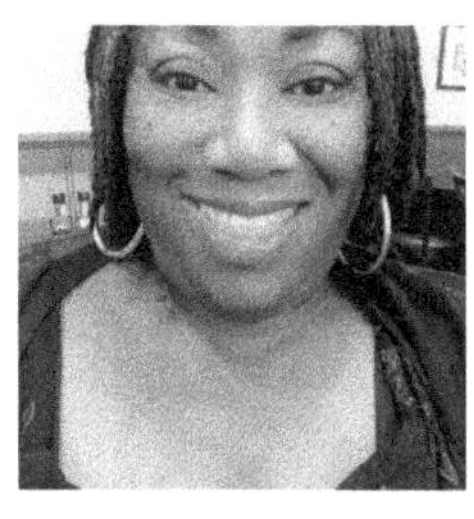

Kathy M. Henry was born in Chicago and she has been writing since she was ten-years-old. She loves to read and writing is an outlet for her vivid imagination. Her motivation for writing is to inform, entertain and hopefully, make people think critically about issues that are affecting society. Although feminism has a bad reputation in current mainstream society, she considers herself to be a feminist who believes in equality for all, not just for a privileged few. She currently resides in Chicago, IL with her children and the fat, black kitty named Diddy.